Lesbian Sperm Tales

BY

Molly Miller

Bloomington, IN 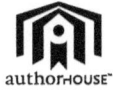 Milton Keynes, UK

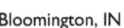

authorHOUSE™

AuthorHouse™
1663 Liberty Drive, Suite 200
Bloomington, IN 47403
www.authorhouse.com
Phone: 1-800-839-8640

AuthorHouse™ UK Ltd.
500 Avebury Boulevard
Central Milton Keynes, MK9 2BE
www.authorhouse.co.uk
Phone: 08001974150

This book is a work of non-fiction. Unless otherwise noted, the author and the publisher make no explicit guarantees as to the accuracy of the information contained in this book and in some cases, names of people and places have been altered to protect their privacy.

First published by AuthorHouse 4/3/2006

ISBN: 1-4259-0544-7 (sc)

Printed in the United States of America
Bloomington, Indiana

This book is printed on acid-free paper.

ACKNOWLEDGMENT

I would like to acknowledge first and foremost my partner, without whose patience, care, and understanding I wouldn't have had the opportunity to experience the best things in life and those yet to come. Our child has enlightened us in enumerable ways and we embrace the opportunities, challenges, and laughter that parenthood affords. Suzanne and Janice, thanks for always being there to listen. Matt, thanks for calling to check on me. Both Cathy and Barbara provided valuable support and guidance we both deeply appreciated. I would also like to thank my uncle whom my son is named after for being my mentor through life; and finally my mom, who is a wonderful grandma. I would also like to thank all the Catholics in our lives that prayed for us during delivery. In today's world, it seems that they were the only ones that were not afraid to use the word "prayer." For everyone else, it was "I'll be thinking about you" or "You will be in my thoughts."

FOREWORD

This novel is not an attempt to disseminate legal, mental health, and/or medical advice. It is simply an attempt to shed light on topics to think about, situations that may be encountered, and above all a plea to put your child first when making decisions. It's not an all-encompassing attempt at trying to capture the very scope of lesbian pregnancy and parenting. It is simply a commentary on our experiences and those of whom we met along the way. Take it for what it is worth: someone's tale of a remarkable event.

INTRODUCTION

If I heard it once, I heard it a thousand times in the weeks and especially the days leading up to the birth of our child. It was repeated in various tones, sentiments, and timbres: "Your life is going to change forever," "You better get all the rest you can now, because you won't when you bring the baby home," and my personal favorite, "Only 'x' amount of days left!" Most of these comments were from people currently parenting, many of whom had walked the newborn path and had experienced all the joy and sleeplessness that follow you home from the hospital. And then the usual suspects fire away with "Are you nervous?" "Are you excited?" or "Why are you so calm? Why aren't you crying?" (That is from those who know that I cry at baseball movies, so the birth of a child should definitely turn on the faucets). For first-time parents, I think the responses to all of these questions should vary. Most of the feelings leading up to the birth are conflicted and happen from moment to moment, day to day, doctor appointment to doctor appointment, fetal heartbeat to ultrasound. If you don't have anything to refer to, compare it to, or even relate it to, then it's hard to get your arms around—these statements about "your life is going to change forever." Now, winning the lottery, I could understand; I can even imagine how I would invest or give the money away. Being responsible for bringing another life into this world, and supporting, nurturing, and most important, loving a child cannot possibly be fathomed until you actually experience it. For lesbian parents, we experience the same fear, doubts, and excitement as heterosexual couples. However, we also have some unique experiences that are germane to the choices we make as lesbian parents.

CHOOSING A FERTILITY CLINIC

Depending on what part of the country in which you live in, people's attitudes, prejudices, and tolerance may be a very important issue to explore. We decided to seek the advice of our OB/GYN on a fertility clinic to go to, as well as the name of a physician to talk with. Later we overheard the receptionist's conversation with an inquiring caller and found that the other physicians in the practice did not inseminate unmarried couples. In fact, the receptionist informed them that the doctor may need to see their marriage certificate at the beginning of the first appointment. My partner and I looked at each other in amazement as we overheard this conversation (and considering HIPAA privacy laws). I just couldn't believe in this day and age that physicians were even discriminatory against single women seeking fertility treatment, let alone lesbians. The caller went on to explain that they wanted to meet with the doctor now; that they were going to get married in a few weeks but already knew they were going to have difficulty conceiving. Again, the receptionist stated that there were other doctors in the practice that would see them but the doctor they were requesting to meet would not see them until after they were married and could provide appropriate documentation. The first meeting with our physician went very well; she asked a few questions, informed us of the mandatory counseling session we had to attend, and then asked us if we wanted to search through their catalogs there at the office to find a donor. My partner and I had already done the research, knew that the clinic worked with four sperm banks, and had already begun the donor search. That is another good question to ask. What sperm banks does the fertility clinic work with? This is important for several reasons, but one personal reason I will share. My partner and I were fortunate enough to have another lesbian couple undergoing the same process we were at the same time only in another state. If it were possible, I think that every couple should find someone that they know and try to go through the process together. This gives everyone someone to talk with, identify with, and later on, to bitch to, if so needed.

The Human Rights Campaign Web site has useful information on "Questions to Ask Before Choosing a Sperm Bank." The information speaks to sperm bank accreditation, screening procedures, fees associated with donor insemination, and other useful information. After deciding on a fertility clinic and exploring sperm banks that work with the fertility clinic, there is also another option that could be explored. There are basically two different types of conception methods available to us lesbians, outside of the traditional "I guess I can sleep with my old boyfriend" method. The more practical methods that you and your partner may agree on are intrauterine insemination, which is performed in the doctor's office, and intracervical insemination, which can be performed at home. Each has its own risks, benefits, and costs. For example, the "at-home" method (also referred to as the turkey-baster method) is less expensive, you can choose your own environment, and you may feel more comfortable than in the sterile environment of a doctor's office. My partner and I chose to go with the intrauterine method and the sterile environment of the doctor's office. It is important to note that women are inseminated when they ovulate, which is determined by an ovulation kit they suggest you purchase and have on hand. The prime opportunity in which to conceive is a narrow opportunity, and this method always feels last minute. Your ordering the sperm and having it shipped to the doctor, you are scheduling an appointment within the next few days, etc. It feels very rushed. You're also rearranging both you and your partner's work schedules, or making up excuses to your co-workers and your boss about why you are calling in sick or canceling meetings or your lunch break ran over two hours. After the first insemination, our process was expedited with a signed consent to have the sperm already thawed when we arrived, instead of the donor's contribution thawing for close to an hour while we wait. Given the unpredictability of ovulation, you may not always have the same nurse available to do the actual insemination. We had someone different each time we went. The entire procedure takes less than ten minutes. (Sound familiar?) However, it was recommended that we wait fifteen to twenty minutes before leaving the office to give ample swim time. We used this time to our advantage, and I would read short excerpts from books about our child's culture and heritage.

DECIDING ON A DONOR

I can only speak about using an anonymous donor. Yes, we talked about using a known donor and other variations, but when it came down to it, it was way too complicated. So we started the process of looking at potential Paternal Genetic Contributors (PGC). The first thing that you need to do is find out what sperm banks your fertility clinic works with. If the clinic works with a bank that is located in your state, chances are you will be looking at lower costs, if you want to consider that. It was tough for me to adjust to the fact that you could potentially look at donors in the privacy of your own home, office, or wherever you have an Internet connection. There was something about choosing a sperm donor online that made me uneasy. I mean there was no indication that they were given personality tests; that they weren't somehow related to Jeffery Dahmer. My partner, who, thank goodness, understands my OCD behavior, continued to laugh with me and let me find my own way through the system. The clinic itself usually has catalogs in their office you can browse through, kind of like Christmas shopping from the Sears or JC Penny catalog.

I suggest making the process fun. After all, you and your partner are making some of the most serious decisions you will ever make in your life; so in light of difficult decision-making, I would suggest that you make the process as fun as possible. This is supposed to be fun, right? We chose to go through the process in the comfort of our own back yard, where we make all of our decisions. I am the "organizer" in the relationship, so I devised a system to at least get us started. We separated potential PGCs into file folders according to the sperm bank that our clinic worked with. A couple of legal pads, Post-it notes, highlighters, and we were in business. Then we added the good stuff. Since "your life is going to change," you might as well start beginning to have a little fun with this important but somewhat stressful event. Choose several evenings, or mornings. There is no way to begin to delve into the numerous potential PGCs in one, two, or three sittings. At the suggestion of our counselor, we started talking with one another about what we "must have" versus "would like to have" in our donor.

As mentioned earlier, choosing a donor profile takes time, patience, and perseverance. During the process of donor selection, we were making a five-hour road trip to see our best friend. This was definitely uninterrupted, continuous time to review the profiles while riding in the car. We had all the necessary materials: highlighter, legal pad, pen, etc. As we were reviewing a donor profile, it dawned on us that our friends (residing in a different state) might be using the same sperm bank. We called them, and sure enough their fertility clinic only worked with one sperm bank, which happened to be one of our four. This particular sperm bank gave basic information over the Internet, and if you wanted an in-depth donor profile, you could pay a nominal fee and they would send it to you. So when we called, we were just checking with them about their experience thus far and to see if they had any extended profiles, etc. Little did we both know we were both looking at the same baby's daddy. However, through the weeding-out process, the donor was tossed; it was still amazing to all of us that we were even entertaining the same donor out of thousands to choose from. Out of hundreds, possibly thousands of donors, we had both chosen the same donor. The odds of this happening are astronomical. After picking our jaws up from the floor of our car, we proceeded to ask some questions, realizing that we didn't want the same donor, as that would just be too weird and the makings for a *Jerry Springer* episode.

Have a number two, or backup donor, in the event that after numerous tries you're not getting pregnant. This is a hard choice. No one likes to think she got pregnant on her number-two choice for a donor. The reality is that God works in mysterious ways, ways we can't always control. I highly recommend shredding ALL but your donor's profile. In other words, if you are like us, you killed a small forest printing out profiles of donors. You have highlighted them, underlined them, numbered them, prioritized them, spilled cheap wine on them, etc. I didn't want our child to ever find other donor profiles while rummaging through my drawers one day. My partner viewed it differently; she said that he might feel like he was chosen over everyone else. The glass is always half full with her; that's what makes her so great.

My partner and I also set a spending limit on the process. For example, we said we were going to try X number of times, which will cost X amount of dollars for X number of months. Costs associated with one insemination include purchasing and shipping the sperm, and the actual insemination itself. The location of the sperm bank will greatly affect your shipping and handling costs. Although we didn't use this as criteria, it was something to consider. For example, you and your partner can agree to try for three months, take three months off to save some money, etc., and then try again for another three months. It was important to me that we have a child, but I didn't want to go bankrupt in the process, especially knowing that raising our child wasn't even going to hold a financial dollar to the cost of conception. I recently read an article that stated that it costs a quarter of a million dollars to raise a child; if everyone knew that, people would be freaking out more. No one can afford to have children, but you can be responsible about your own future. Until you do, do plan carefully.

A good question to ask yourselves is do you see either one of you having additional children in the future, and if so, would you want your child to be genetically related. If your answer is yes, you would want your children to be genetically related, then you will want to investigate the number of sperm vials available for purchase and if the donor is a regular contributor or if they have retired from donating sperm. If there are remaining vials left to purchase, the next step would be to investigate having them stored appropriately until you are both ready to conceive another child. Both the fertility clinics and sperm banks have information on storage.

There are both disadvantages and advantages to choosing an unknown donor. Although sperm banks are regimented in their screening and testing process, they also abide by federal and state laws. Researching the sperm banks' testing and screening processes is highly recommended, and information usually is found on their Web sites or by calling them as well.

If you choose mornings as your review time, go out for coffee, sit outside at a café, or sit inside on a cold morning around a fireplace in your local coffee shop. Go easy on yourself and reduce the pressure by putting some time limits around each "review session." This will keep both of you from going crazy. We frequently chose the evening, as it was after work and seasonally the weather in early summer in the Midwest is beautiful. It was not uncommon for us to fire up the Chimneas and line the edge of our patio with torches. (After a while it was beginning to look like a runway and we became fearful of airplanes landing in our back yard.) We would often choose some music and then for the finale would add a wine-and-cheese plate. And let's not forget the office supplies I mentioned earlier! We would use the method that was recommended by our counselor and start off with two columns: "would like to have" and "must have."

A one-hour counseling session was mandated by the fertility clinic that we used. We wouldn't do this every evening, but knew we would like to narrow our selection process down and have the first insemination within a few months of beginning the process. From hundreds we narrowed it down rapidly within a few weeks and had our winner.

In looking at several donor qualities, it was important to us to look at where we were right then and where we were going in the future. For example, we had two dogs and a cat when we were choosing a donor, so it was important for us to have it noted either that the donor didn't have any pet allergies or, if that question wasn't asked, we looked to see if they currently had pets or had been raised with pets. Other information including the donor's favorite sports, hobbies, and education may be available. Different sperm banks collect different types of information and have diverse types of histories that may be of interest in making your decision. Again, sometimes there are additional fees associated with requesting added information about the donor outside of the profile they typically provide. Basically, allow yourself and your partner time, space, freedom of expression and emotion, and most important, know when to say "uncle." Know when you need to take a break, stop for the day, and stop for the week.

Usually, clinics may recommend X number of inseminations with the same donor sperm, and if unsuccessful may suggest going to another selection before looking at other medical options that may be interfering with conception. Lesbians that I have talked with do get disappointed when they are not pregnant on the first try. Here are a few tips that have helped lesbians; although not medically proven they have been tried and true. First and foremost, be patient with the process; carefully choose the "brand" of ovulation kit; have sex the night before the insemination; and take your partner with you on the appointment, if you are in a relationship (I would consider this a must, but some don't), or if single, take a trusted friend. The insemination process is not the most romantic and is actually quite quick and mechanical in nature. Personally, we thought the best part of the "insemination" appointment was the short time prior to the actual procedure, when you had the opportunity to pick up or hold the vial of sperm. (I was shocked to find that the vial was clear, tinted with pink—that wasn't how I remembered it!) In our case, we picked up the vial, and we took turns holding it, which kept it warm while we walked down the hall to the doctor's office. The actual procedure took less than ten minutes. I was told by several people that I could actually inject the sperm into my partner after the nurse had placed the tip of the syringe at the top of her cervix. It is suggested that you speak with your doctor and/or check your state's donor insemination law. I chose not to pursue this option because when my partner was pregnant or while she was in the process of delivery, I didn't want her to be able to say, "You did this to me!" After the injection of the sperm, it is recommended that the person continue lying down for the next approximately twenty minutes. After a few unsuccessful attempts at conceiving, we chose this time to do something unique instead of staring at each other, glancing at our watches. We chose to get some books about our soon-to-be child's heritage and ethnicity, and while we were waiting out our twenty minutes, I read to her. It could just be that we are quirky, but after trying some different things and relaxing a little bit more, conception soon followed.

FAMILY MEDICAL LEAVE ACT AND OUTING YOURSELF AT WORK

Okay, you're happy, you're partner's happy, you're pregnant—now what? Before picking out a paint color and a theme for the nursery, I decided to panic about FMLA and how I was going to access leave from work. FMLA is very clear about who is eligible to take it and how it protects people who access it. For example, I was pursuing adoption of our child, so therefore I was eligible to access FMLA; in a state where second-parent adoption is prohibited, I wouldn't be eligible to access FMLA or be protected by it.

Basically, the Family Medical Leave Act (FMLA) grants eligible employees (please refer to your employers personnel policy handbook and/or the Department of Labor specifics) twelve weeks of unpaid leave during a twelve-month period of time for certain qualifying reasons. Pursuing adoption is considered a reason to access FMLA. I highly suggest if you are seeking a second-parent adoption that you speak with your attorney as well as a representative of your employer's human resources department. This is usually a unique situation and most likely they may not know exactly how to respond; in my case, I was told, "I haven't done one of those yet." Company policy varies widely regarding how they implement FMLA beyond the minimum the federal law dictates. Accessing FMLA affords the employee certain rights and protections, many of which your immediate supervisor may not be aware of. Explore your company's policy regarding the use of paid leave, vacation leave, sick leave, or a combination thereof. I had to submit the final petition of adoption to my employer for documentation of my leave. I discovered that my immediate supervisor knew very little of the FMLA provisions or its entitlements, which left me in a position to educate not only myself but others as well. I strongly encourage you to investigate your company's policy regarding accessing FMLA benefits, whether you are seeking a second-parent adoption or you are the partner giving birth.

Along with exploring your company's FMLA policy, and if you choose to access the leave or even if you take an extended leave from work to care for your son or daughter, you will most likely be faced with a lot of questions, especially if you are not the one who is pregnant. For example, you may have a position in which planning certain events and/or activities is part of your job, so that "certain" times of the year, you know job responsibilities take precedent over vacation time. However, during the course of family planning, you and your partner are having your child during one of these "forbidden" periods. You may find yourself in a situation in which you not only may be coming out but you also may find yourself adding that you are also expecting a child. These situations can be disconcerting if you are not prepared or do not know what to anticipate. I was never ashamed of my family situation or to acknowledge our new plans. However, I always had this philosophy: people usually don't introduce themselves to me as "straight," so why should I introduce myself to others as a "lesbian"? It's what I am, not who I am. Others may share a different view and that is perfectly fine; most of our friends certainly do.

SUPPORTING THE NON-PREGNANT PARTNER

During the next nine months, all—and I mean ALL—of the focus is on your pregnant partner. It is time to get used to being number two, and if you're fortunate you won't slip below the rank of your once-all-encompassing canine and feline friends. The glowing "mom-to-be" gets all the attention; questions are always directed to her such as "When are you due?" "How far along are you?" and "Have you picked out any names?" etc. Meanwhile, being the type B personality my partner is, she answered all the questions. In the beginning, it's tough to understand that you're not necessarily being "excluded," but not "included" either. It's not uncommon to feel a little kicked to the curb. The NPP is doing all the grunt work, rivaling the efforts of a Sherpa making the final push for the summit on Mount Everest.

After the birth there are other things to contend with that add to being left out of the experience. Everyone is constantly commenting on how the child looks like the birth mother. No kidding. Although that is true for many obvious reasons, it can pull at the heartstrings. For me it was a constant reminder that I didn't contribute biologically to our child, and that being lesbians we weren't capable of producing a child ourselves. Have a friend that you can confide in, talk, laugh, and cry with. It will help the process go so much more smoothly when you feel you can address your insecurities and most important, be yourself.

THE PARTNER'S NIGHTMARE

You will gain weight. My partner was forbidden to gain weight, although she did, but ate better when she was pregnant than when she wasn't. If she gained a pound it was due to consuming an orange, vegetables, nutrition bars, and the like. I felt as if we were living in Southern California. I, however, put on every pound related to pregnancy that she didn't. In retrospect, I guess I felt bad for her or thought I would use the excuse myself to eat pints of ice cream, greasy pizzas, and cheeseburgers. I was the epitome of sympathy eating. She even came out of the hospital after giving birth weighing less than she did before she was pregnant. Not me: I managed to put on twenty pounds. Now my treadmill is a coat rack and I am still fat.

If gaining excess weight isn't enough, because we are women I became subjected to what felt like a study in human pheromones. It is no mystery that husbands, partners, etc., experience a variety of pregnancy symptoms; entire books are dedicated to the human mystery. For instance, once my partner was pregnant, my menstrual cycle changed completely. I noticed within the first two weeks, in fact, that it had changed dramatically. In the two weeks following the insemination, prior to the at-home pregnancy test, I told her that she was pregnant based on my bodily symptoms. She had always been the alpha dog, even in pregnancy. Now I know that this may seem a bit farfetched, and in some relationships it may be. After fifteen years, I think I know her and I know my body. After she was pregnant, my twenty-eight-day cycle turned into twenty-two, thirty-six—hell, I even skipped a month (which had NEVER happened). Be forewarned: they are painful, long, heavy, and horrible; at times I wished I either was pregnant myself or was begging for a hysterectomy. I talked to our fertility doctor about this "menstrual synchrony" and "pheromone phenomenon." I was quickly dismissed. I used the archaic "college dorm" example that often occurs when women live in close quarters. This phenomenon was first described in 1971 by researcher Martha McClintock of the University of Chicago. In California, at the Sonoma State Hospital Brain Behavior Research Center, scientists identified what they termed "menstrual pacesetters"; they made other women conform to their cycles. If your pregnant partner is a menstrual pacesetter, or alpha dog—call them what you want—your body can change. Penn State physician Robert Heinbach shares in his research that "pheromones are chemical messages passed between members of species, which are odorless but are picked up by our sense of smell or olfactory nervous system." I share this only because it happened to me. I would recommend seeing a gynecologist if you become concerned. Funny, after my partner stopped breastfeeding, I returned to normal, like clockwork. I now owned by body again after almost a year. What the NPP needs is a little reassurance that she is not crazy; that her body will come back when her partner does.

<u>LAST TIMES</u>

After the "last times," "getting all the rest you can," "doing the rocket launch countdown," "anticipating the next or any type of nervous breakdown," you find that the few days prior to the birth (in our case we knew the scheduled day because she was having a Cesarean section) all you really do is sit around and stare at each other. The "new sense of calmness" that is referenced in the book *What to Expect When You're Expecting* comes back around, thank goodness. Maybe it's denial; maybe it's your body and mind's way of preparing yourself that is far away from the recesses of your mind. Maybe it's the acceptance of reality or the realization that you can't turn back so you might as well "take one for the team and buck up." Who knows…. I'll tell you in a few days. This brief, albeit comical, account of our pregnancy and impending birth needs to begin before our delivery. Why? Because "my life is going to change forever!" Our best friend has two children; we all met in college and therefore have quite a history. Anyone you spent your twenty-first birthday and shared a toilet with can probably get you both through the birth of your child. The only downfall is that she has us in this space of arrested development, as if we have never behaviorally matured and therefore still problem solve as though we were in our early twenties, not late thirties. With all that aside, she has been lovely. I say that before I lead into the fact that she called me every morning around 6:30 a.m. with the following phrase: "Only four more days. Why aren't you crying yet?" Not allowing me to respond, day after day, week after week of this, she simply has now begun stating, "Well, they must have increased your meds," as if I am a schizophrenic on Ativan and I will start hallucinating at any minute. I continue to respond that I cannot "will" my body into total freak-out mode, and who has time for that anyway? With two screaming kids in the background, I can't call her. Every time I need support, I call; she says the same thing (at a whisper): "Let me call you back in a few minutes." Are you kidding? It's always a few fucking days; by that time, I have indulged in a mind-numbing lesbian romance book, popped the cork on an inexpensive Chardonnay, watched a very predictable Lifetime movie, and sucked it up. Just for kicks, I always ask her why she is whispering, just to see what she says. After four years of thinking I need a hearing aid when I talk to her, I now wanted to see if she had come up with a new reason. No, not really; it's the same ones: one or both boys are sleeping, one is eating, one is in the bath, my husband just got home, the cat is looking at me funny, etc.... My partner and I, after four years of this, have made a Girl Scout and Brownie (she didn't make it to the Scouts) promise that there will be ABSOLUTELY NO FUCKING WHISPERING IN OUR HOUSE. Not that we don't know the difference between our indoor and outdoor voices, but get real, people; I can't press my phone any harder against my head to try to hear her before I have Sony emblazoned on my earlobe!

SUPPORT SYSTEMS

We have established that it is critical to have a support person(s), preferably people that know you fairly well and who can tolerate you saying things you don't really mean and having all the symptoms of a pregnant person, except you're not the one who is pregnant. Oh yeah, I forgot the best phrase I have come to learn from our dear friend: "You'll understand once you have kids of your own." As if we are just dumb-asses until that point! Oh, that's right; my life is going to change forever. How quickly one forgets!

HELPING THE NON-PREGNANT ONE THROUGH THE NEXT NINE MONTHS

Many books are dedicated to the pregnant woman; most include paragraphs and often commit chapters to the father. As women we experience the pregnancy much differently than if we were playing the role of doting fathers. After experiencing potential menstrual cycle changes, and dealing with the lack of attention that the pregnant partner is receiving, we are often left searching for our support system and pleading for understanding. The following chapter is dedicated to the pregnant partner and how she can help support the process. Understand that even though we are not the ones giving birth, we are sharing some very major concerns. These concerns are for the health of the partner as well as the baby. We share the same uncertainty about parenting. Not about the choice of having a baby, but about raising a baby to be a happy, healthy, and secure adult. We are concerned about taking time off from our jobs, about daycare, and providing financial security. We are also exhausted at the end of the day; we have put in our eight hours and assumed a great amount of additional responsibility around the house, and willingly. We are trying to meet all of your needs and still take care of ourselves. We are excited, hesitant, and scared. We are frightened about the rights we will have as a second parent in a same-sex relationship. If we are not already thoroughly exhausted, we also assume the role of caretaker in other ways.

Partner "to-do" list (approx 1-2 weeks prior to birth)

- Mow the lawn (if seasonally and environmentally appropriate).
- Bag of dog food or cat food; or, if you are unfortunate to have both, make sure you have a bag of each. You don't need a hungry pet and a hungry infant.
- Change the air filter in your furnace.
- Change the oil in both cars. (I didn't find this helpful tidbit in any book I read; chances are one or both of you are in need of an oil change, so

why not have both cars serviced prior to delivery? One less thing to worry about.)

- Think about where your pregnant partner would really like to go out to eat. Either make reservations or go early; believe me, they are in no shape this late in pregnancy to wait in line.

- Review the checklist in *What to Expect When You're Expecting*; get what you need and some things that you don't.

- Make sure you have a centralized place and receptacle for any and all receipts.

- Send an e-mail to those that will be either participating in the birthing experience or traveling, outlining any of the "rules" that have been set forth by you and your partner under the guise of doctor's orders and/or hospital rules.

- Regardless of the "type" of birthing experience, pack a snack bag, including your favorite beverage; both you and your partner will appreciate it, especially if the hospital cafeteria is under construction or closed.

- Make sure you have someone to house-sit your pets or make kennel reservations. (If your baby is due during a peak travel season such as spring break or Thanksgiving, make sure you make your reservations in advance; most urban and suburban kennels with outstanding reputations fill up months in advance.)

- Although dreary and drab, you need at least two copies of your legal papers (one that you will take to the hospital and one to give to the OB to send to the maternity ward to have in your partner's medical records). This should include at a minimum: your partner's living will, healthcare power of attorney, durable power of attorney, legal guardianship for your partner, and legal guardianship for your child. True enough, this often is viewed as an extra burden and an added expense, especially when you are thinking about diapers, formula, breast pumps, and daycare. However, you can't put a price tag on the safety and rights of your child and your partner. See a lawyer for estimates and set aside anywhere between 650 and 1,200 bucks. Hey, if you are responsible enough to bring a child into this world then you need to take care of first things first. Now is the time to get your priorities straight, not later!

FINAL DAYS

The final days approaching the birth are filled with "last time." This was a common phrase uttered by my partner and me for weeks before our child was born, at times jokingly and at times lamenting our responsibility. This is the last time we will be eating lunch out as a couple and not "parents." This is the last Friday before I become a parent. This is the last time I will be able to take a bath while indulging in a great book and treating myself to a glass of wine. What I didn't know was that last year's Mother's Day was the last one I would spend as only a daughter. Upon reflection, that is mind blowing. During the last week, we covered the mundane to the ridiculous; we believed that one of the greatest qualities we could bring to parenting was our ability to laugh at ourselves, both individually and as a couple. Then there is the overwhelming desire to prepare your lives for the storm of the century that is heading your way. Why else would anyone in one weekend buy forty pounds worth of dog food, five pounds of dog bones, three cases of soda, change the oil in the car, replace the air filter in the furnace, mow the lawn, and then decide to … as if any of these things cannot be accomplished once you have the baby!

I had a few critical moments during the pregnancy and birth of our child. One of the most memorable, besides the birth of our child, was a phone call I received the night before we were scheduled to deliver. I had an old high school and college friend that I had recently reconnected with the year before, after finding her e-mail address through college reunion materials. After losing contact for several years, we reconnected through e-mail and even managed to get together for a WNBA game that summer. We had known each other since seventh grade, and yes, she does know where the bodies are buried! Actually, my partner's first day of insemination was the night of the

WNBA game. During the next year, I informed her of our pregnancy and progress, etc. The night before our child was born, she called me not knowing that the actual day of delivery was within the next twenty-four hours. She called to see how I was holding up and I blew her away with the timing of her call. Then it was her turn to blow me away. She told me to hang on; that there was someone that wanted to speak with me. The person got on the phone and began idle chitchat, etc. I had to admit I didn't recognize the voice. It was my high school coach, whom I hadn't seen or spoken with in over twenty years. When you are consumed with fear and doubt, elated but scared out of your mind, fearful but happy, etc., who do you need to talk with to get you through the next twenty-four hours? Your coach. I highly recommend, if you have a relationship, either current or past, reestablishing this connection for this primary purpose. There are things that are so primal that only a coach can know. I don't even think that they know it, but they will give you the confidence that you may be lacking. That conversation was worth its weight in gold and will never be forgotten. In summary, your support system should include people that know you better than you know yourself, for those unsuspecting moments that you need support but are unaware of it.

SEEKING
SECOND-PARENT ADOPTION

The Human Rights Campaign Web site *http://www.hrc.org* has a wealth of information regarding state adoption laws. The Human Rights Campaign Web site also contains information on state custody and visitation laws as well as donor insemination laws. The state-specific information includes whether or not single GLBT individuals are permitted to petition to adopt, same-sex couples jointly petitioning for adoption, as well as information on state laws permitting a same-sex partner to petition to adopt a partner's adopted child. Sound confusing? It is. Some states only allow certain adoptions and certain counties within a state may permit only certain types of adoptions. It can get overwhelming and exhausting. There are as many laws regarding adoption as there are states. I would recommend locating an attorney that is familiar with same-sex adoption proceedings in your state. When meeting your attorney, ask questions regarding the number of adoptions she or he has done, the paperwork needed, any potential legislative changes that might occur prior to the adoption, and the costs associated with the adoption process. Fees associated with the adoption process vary widely and can be upwards of $3,000 to $4,000. Specifically, fees that may vary from state to state include legal fees, filing fees, putative father registry, and adoption history fees. The process also requires that an adoption summary or home study be completed, and there are costs associated with this depending on if you have it done privately or after you file your petition to adopt. In some states, that fee will be considerably lower if you are seeking a special-needs adoption. Seeking adoption assures that your child will have the same rights heterosexual couples have; for instance, entitlement to death benefits, etc. If pursuing adoption is not an option ONLY because your state prohibits it, you may want to pursue legal guardianship as a measure to at least ensure some legal rights for your place in the child's life to make legal decisions, etc. Seeking second-parent adoption protects the rights of your child, an avenue that should be pursued. If second-parent adoption is not prohibited in your state but your partner has reservations about you adopting "her" child, I would suggest taking a good look at the joint decision that you both made as well as seek couples' counseling. There are other things to consider as well, including a name change. If your petition is granted, you may have the option of the entire family changing their last name, so that all of you share the same last name; or you can keep it the same as the birth mother's or choose to hyphenate your last name, in which case the birth mother's last name will be last. I can't stress enough the importance of beginning to explore this process once you both learn of the pregnancy. Again, the legal proceedings are about protecting the rights of your child, bar none.

Depending on state law, it may take upwards of sixty to ninety days before you receive a court date. Your attorney can file the petition for adoption once your child is born. Your attorney may need specific information for the petition such as the name of child, gender, length, weight, date, and time of birth, etc. In some states there is a specified waiting period after the petition is filed; your attorney will know the state-specific information.

Once you receive the date for your adoption hearing, ask if cameras are permitted. Even a disposable one will work to capture the moment. Also, please take your baby, the grandparents, etc.; this is a major day. My son talked or babbled through most of my testimony and that of my partners, and we didn't know whether to giggle silently (after all, we were in a courtroom) or have one of us take him outside the courtroom. He remained, and after our testimony was over the judge asked our attorney if there were any other comments, etc., regarding the adoption petition. She replied, "Yes, but I think he is too young to testify"! It was a comical moment in the courtroom, a much-needed tension reliever!

After my petition for second-parent adoption was granted, we rejoiced in the aftermath of what seemed like an arduous year in preparation, waiting, and wondering. The clerk of courts handed us a piece of paper; she said it was for our baby's book. We didn't look at it at the time; we were getting copies of the adoption paperwork, talking, taking pictures with the judge, etc. That evening when we got home, we pulled out the paperwork and read the following:

LEGACY OF AN ADOPTED CHILD

Once there were two women. Two different lives shaped to make you one. One became your guiding star; the other became your sun. The first one gave you life, and the second taught you to live it. The first gave you a need for love. The second was there to give it. One gave you nationality. The other gave you a new name.

One gave you talent. The other gave you aim. One gave you emotions. The other calmed your fears. One saw your first sweet smile. The other dried your tears. One sought for you a home that she could not provide. The other prayed for a child, and her hope was not denied.

And now you ask, through your tears, the age-old question; unanswered through the years: Heredity or Environment—which are you a product of?

Neither my child. Neither.
Just two different kinds of love.

Author unknown

ASSIGNING GUARDIANSHIP POST BIRTH—(things to think about)

Now that the hard part is over, you both are parents and learning the trials and tribulations of parenthood. Do not postpone the assignment of guardianship should something happen to your partner or both of you. Usually, the first person you think of is also someone you spend a lot of time with. Not to be grim, but think of a second and, to be on the safe side, a third designated guardian. It's a tough conversation to have with your partner, but it is in the best interest of your child(ren). A question that I have heard people raise is, should the guardian of our child be gay or not? That is an individual question that couples/families will have to ask themselves. For us, we looked at family values, stability, similar views on work and education, faith, etc. We arrived at our conclusion by determining who would raise our child in the most similar environment with as much love, and who shared our values. For us, sexual orientation didn't enter into the evaluation process.

CHOOSING A DAYCARE

Start early. For my partner and me it was important that we had our son in a daycare that was okay with him having two mommies. In order to achieve this objective without cold-calling daycares and inquiring about the obvious, I decided this was a prime opportunity to do some networking with other gays and lesbians. I e-mailed and called others who might know someone that might know someone else, etc., letting them know I was looking for daycare that was gay friendly. Within a few days I had an interview scheduled for both of us at a daycare that at least met our initial and most important needs. I have it on good authority from those that I know in the daycare business that initially inquiring about whether or not they are "okay" with the two-mom thing will result in a resounding "sure" and a puzzled, quizzical look. "Sure" equals an application fee (which is non-refundable), and every daycare is a business. So it is important to thoroughly investigate the daycare, take a tour, meet the director, and introduce yourself to the person(s) who will be caring for your infant. We were also surprised to find out that "part-time" daycare is not that easy to find. We also knew that Grandma would be picking our son up from daycare, so we scheduled an appointment for Grandma to see the daycare and meet the staff prior to our son's first day. Grandma felt better having met everyone, and isn't that what it is all about—making Grandma feel better?

HOSPITAL BAG

My partner did not, despite what she says, do one bit of "nesting," so do not put off pulling together the hospital bag.

1. Prepaid phone card: You are prohibited from using cell phones in hospitals, so unless you are planning an at-home delivery, this may be a smart purchase. I found that I didn't want to leave the room for extended periods of time to go outside and use my cell phone to call people.

2. Playing cards: You won't need these for a C-section, but I surmise that you will need them for a vaginal birth, if there is a lot of waiting. Despite my partner having a C-section, I brought a regular deck of cards, UNO, Crazy 8's, Old Maid, and Seven-card Stud for Dummies. Now, we were only in the hospital for forty-eight hours, so we didn't get a chance to use these, but they came in handy at home during recuperation.

3. Snack foods and beverages: Pack some light snacks: peanuts, pretzels, candy bars, nutrition/breakfast bars, etc. Our hospital's cafeteria was under construction, which became my worst nightmare when I found the time to eat. And it goes without saying how wonderful hospital food is. I also brought some water and pop so I could avoid trying to find vending machines.

4. Laptop: Some hospitals may permit the use of laptop computers so that you can upload digital photos of the new bundle of joy and send them out.

5. Cameras: Most people are shooting with digital cameras these days. I am from the old school and used a 35 mm to shoot the birth of our child (with automatic focus; you won't have time to focus or steady the hands). Also, our doctor was willing to take our first "family" picture in the OR. Imagine the surprise on our doctor's face when I handed her my camera and expected her to know how to use it and not mess up the one opportunity we had to have this shot. So, being

ultra-prepared, I whipped out a disposable, high-definition camera with flash, with which no one—not even an MD—can take a bad picture! There isn't a lot of time, and I was grateful she was willing to do it, so I wanted to make it easy for her.

6. Most important, please bring copies of all your essential documents, including power of attorney, living will, and legal guardianship documents.

7. If you have pets, make sure you have made arrangements for their care while both of you are at the hospital. During peak vacation times, many kennels book months if not a year in advance. If you know the due date, and will need to board your pets during your hospital stay, make sure and get on their radar screen.

8. If you have someone house-sitting your pets, and are able to come home for a few hours each day, many recommend bringing home some of the baby's blankets so that the dogs/cats can smell the person that they will be second in command to. Our pets didn't really pay that much attention to

the blankets I brought home each day; actually, they really didn't notice the baby until he made a noise!

AT THE HOSPITAL

Our doctor was awesome in making some great suggestions to us as a family. Probably the most important suggestion she made was that we should have the first hour alone with our child after the birth, therefore postponing the barrage of "grandparentness" for at least sixty minutes so we could catch our breath, cry in peace, and start breastfeeding without an audience. We even told our parents that the hour after birth was for bonding per doctor's orders. I can't stress this enough, and when you can blame it on the doctor then you and your partner are off the hook. Our hospital allowed the significant other that was staying with the birth mother to spend the nights. Their policy was to also "band" this person with the number associated with the baby as well as with the birth mother's name. This was very useful when they brought the baby back from testing, especially sometimes in the middle of the night, or if the birth mother was showering, etc. They then could match the infant with the partner, therefore not always disturbing the birth mother. It was also a neat way of underscoring the importance of you being the second parent.

You would be fooling yourself if after an eight- or twelve-hour nursing shift was over, when the RNs and LPNs gathered around the nursing station to give reports, that they didn't announce the "lesbians" in room seven. Most are appropriate; I refuse to explain myself during most occasions anyway. It's kind of like they write the capital L on your hospital chart. Be wary, be cautious, be respectful, and most of all, retain your dignity.

BIRTH CERTIFICATE

During your hospital stay, the birth mother will be asked to supply information for the birth certificate. If you want to hyphenate the last name of your child, you will most likely encounter some resistance with the hospital staff. In fact, you may hear a phrase similar to this: "I don't know if we can do that." In reality, you can name your child anything you want. But in our case, we were forewarned by our attorney that this would most likely happen and not to worry, we could change the name at the adoption hearing. In our case, after the nurses gathered around the water cooler and talked with their administrative person that handled birth certificates, they concluded that our request couldn't be granted. I never thought that a punctuation mark would cause such controversy. We thought we would try anyway; in any case, it was an effort on our part to increase their awareness of and sensitivity to same-sex couples. If your petition for second-parent adoption is granted, you can change the name of your child on the birth certificate. However, after the adoption hearing and you receive your new birth certificate in the mail, don't be surprised when the partner is listed as the baby's father.

Another interesting but disturbing factoid is how the birth mother shows up in statewide statistics, specifically under "non-marital births." Kids Count is a national and state-by-state effort to track the status of children in the U.S., a project of the Annie E. Casey Foundation. The goal of collecting this data is to assist with informing local, state, and federal officials in an attempt to secure a better future for children. According to state-specific Kids Count data, the non-marital birth rate in our state has continued to climb. Information concerning the race and age of the birth mother is also collected, and consequently information is derived from this. According to Kids Count 2004, "Children of unmarried mothers are at higher risk of having adverse outcomes such as low birth weight and infant mortality. These children are also more likely to live in poverty because the social, emotional, and financial resources available to the family may be less available than for children of married mothers." I am not going to argue the fact that collection of this data is important and oftentimes drives services and treatment that are much needed by pregnant and parenting mothers. However, I do find it disturbing that my partner has now become one of these statistics that I find inaccurate. She is now documented has having a non-marital birth and has become part of state and national statistics. I am not going to debate the gay marriage issue. However, in my view, my partner should not be part of these statistics because it portrays an inaccurate view of our family. Collection of this data does not allow for nontraditional families giving birth and raising children. We have a long way to go nationally to recognize families of all types; portraying lesbian birth mothers as in these statistics is alarming. Not for one minute did I think that we would fall into one of these high-risk categories; we are raising our child in a two-parent home. Collection of this data also does not allow for the decision of single individuals, gay or straight, whose families are also termed "non-marital births" when in fact single people raise very healthy, well-adjusted children all the time.

OUTLAWS AND GRANDMAS

You animal lovers will just love this one. "What about the dogs? I am afraid they're just not going to know what to do, or will they eat the baby?" Okay, folks, the only thing that eats babies is Fat Bastard from *Austin Powers*. Second, no shit the dogs aren't going to know what to do. Hell, we don't even know what we are doing, and you're expecting a canine to intuitively pick up how to act around a baby? Come on … they're specialties are retrieving tennis balls and taking up too much room in the bed; they didn't go to "new parents having a baby" class.

Be patient with all the grandparents; it is an enormously proud moment for them as well. They have varying concerns about whether the baby is too hot or too cold. They still think that bourbon gum rubs soothe teething and don't know why we go to the expense of disposable diapers. They are baffled and befuddled by car seats, and need educated on SIDS because they can't figure out why the baby isn't lying on its stomach. Diapers even now give gentle reminders—"back to sleep"—which I think is a splendid idea, but help the grandparents with how things have progressed in the last thirty or forty years. In an effort to help inform my mother how things have changed, I recommended that she subscribe to a couple of the numerous e-newsletters that are available to give her minute-by-minute (really, it's week-by-week) child-development information. She has found it tremendously helpful and has now taken it upon herself to give us pointers! It's a great way for grandparents to learn without us barking at them every minute, especially if they are actively involved in the childrearing process.

They may also be rather clueless about why you are pursuing guardianship or adoption, and may not understand why it is important. It's an education process, one with which we need to have patience. Our parents have most likely been raised in a much more traditional society; they may be okay with their child being gay, but introducing a grandchild to the mix requires a special kind of tolerance.

WELCOME-HOME BASKET

I found it helpful, basically to keep myself occupied, to make a welcome-home gift basket for my partner. I have listed below a few things that I included; my goal was to help her feel better about herself after giving birth:

- Crest white strips.
- Tanning package. (La Leche research indicated that if you were breastfeeding and wanted to indoor tan, keep your breasts covered.) This ensured that she could have at least a mandatory twenty minutes outside the house, which she began to look forward to.
- Her favorite lotions and soaps.
- Box of hair color.
- A novel.
- A new, relaxing CD.
- Triple-sheet the bed with linen spray.
- Change a few of the pictures in your house. There are numerous Web sites that offer low-cost, discounted posters that can be self-framed, and this adds a new flair to the home environment.
- Purchase a special frame for those first few pictures; display them in the house before she comes home, if you have the opportunity. Thank

goodness for digital cameras, with which you can print at home and/or at one-hour photo labs.

- Change a few pots that house your favorite plants.

There are numerous other things that could be added, but time is always a factor. You have nine months to put this together, if you think about it. It reminds me of people that do last-minute Christmas shopping on Christmas Eve, often lamenting that they just didn't have the time. Christmas happens every 364 days; it shouldn't be a surprise.

THE FIRST FEW WEEKS

There is nothing that can prepare you for the first few weeks at home. At the recommendation of our OB/GYN, I took off the first two weeks after the birth, and then returned to work. She made a good point, one that we had never thought of. Why have both of you be tired? I returned to work after two weeks, and then took several weeks off when my partner returned to work. This helped in several ways. First, my partner said it was easier returning to work knowing that on her first day back she didn't have to drop the baby off at daycare; and second, this gave me the much-needed time with our child I so desperately craved.

The first few weeks you are at home you will have to get used to some new noises. Of course, the sound of your newborn and every sound cause ultra-alertness and hyper-vigilance. I remember trying to get used to the baby monitors that were in our bedroom and other areas of the house. They always had this dull, static hum. I was waiting for the following phrase to come over the monitors: "Carol Ann, Carol Ann." The static was too reminiscent of the movie *Poltergeist*, in which a family is trying to communicate with their child through a static-ridden television set. A few words of caution about baby monitors: If you partner is in the baby's room, where the receiver is, she will learn that she can talk to you throughout the house wherever the speakers are stationed. When she learned she could communicate with me, I thought (due to lack of sleep, I'm sure) that I could communicate back using the same method. So after being home a few days, my partner was in the baby's room asking me to do a few things, etc. Without giving it any thought, I picked up the receiver in the kitchen and began talking back, like a walkie-talkie. She gently tapped me on my shoulder and said, "I was afraid you were doing that!" Intellectually I knew better, but you temporarily lose your mind without sleep! This was one of the few laughing moments we had had since the birth; we were in desperate need of some comic relief. Conversely, the monitors can also get you into a lot of trouble. Believe me, after a while you will forget they are there, that Carol Ann is inside your monitors, or the power they possess! I mentioned earlier the crucial role that your support system has for both of you. Chances are you may both share some of the same support persons. Be careful how close you are to the baby's room if you happen to be venting your frustrations about your partner to your "support system"!

BREASTFEEDING

There are many well-documented benefits to breast-feeding your child. Your partner may choose to breastfeed over the bottle. I attended the Breastfeeding 101 class with my partner so that I could learn more about how I could help her through the process. The classes usually are not tailored to "two moms," so I really paid attention when they mentioned "dad's role." There is a lot that the NPP can do to contribute to the breastfeeding experience by supporting her partner. I learned in class that I can be of help by getting the baby when he awakes, changing him, and bringing him to her. I also learned how important it was for her to stay hydrated, so I would bring her water while she was feeding. I also logged what I termed the "airline coordinates" for the feeding: "left breast, fifteen minutes." It was suggested that we track this information for a while, but it was comical looking at a page of undecipherable documentation! This is also a time in which the NPP can feel as though she is not bonding with the baby as much as she would like. In other words, the biological mother's role during breastfeeding is crucial;

however, the down side is that the baby is with her in the beginning all the time. It was not until she started using a breast pump that allowed me to bottle-feed that I started to feel just a little more connected. Be patient; this is a wonderful opportunity for the biological mom and the baby to bond, connect, and share this experience. For the NPP, be patient; seize the opportunities that arise when the baby is not feeding, although they are few and far between in the beginning!

FROM BURBERRY TO SPONGEBOB SQUAREPANTS

Okay, with a child comes a few sacrifices. My partner always said we had champagne tastes with a beer pocket book. I had to make a few changes. These changes had to do with hobbies and habits—no surprise there! I started with limiting my Starbucks habit to once or twice a week; the remainder of the week, if I was on the road, it would be gas station coffee. My other habits and hobbies had to cease as well. Understandably, none of these things were that necessary, just nice, when you have the money, to indulge in such things. It doesn't seem like a huge sacrifice; after all, you are bringing into the world a new life, one that will "change" your life forever and make all the sacrifices you ever made seem small or infinitesimal. I also needed to curb my spending habits; although infrequent, I was often indulgent when I did spend. I finally noticed my latest parent fashion statement shortly after our child was born. My partner's work friends wanted to stop over one evening to see the baby and say hello. I was too tired to change and didn't really care what I looked like or what I was wearing. I watched my partner for the first time since we had been home (all of one week) try to pull herself together; you know, blow-dry your hair, put on clothes that weren't wrinkle free or that had been worn the day before. Anyhow, I donned for the visit what I had been wearing all day: my Burberry boxer shorts and a SpongeBob SquarePants T-shirt. Now, let me explain even the possession of the T-shirt, which wouldn't normally grace my wardrobe. A few years ago our best friend was giving birth via C-section to her second child. As we prepared for our weeklong excursion of caring for her, her infant, and a three-year-old toddler, we were trying to think of everything. Knowing her toddler was a big fan of the Sponge, I found a T-shirt sporting the newly popular undersea creature at a discount store and purchased it, thinking that if the toddler threw himself out during my watch I could probably score some points by pointing at my shirt and repeating "SpongeBob" over and over until he quieted down and realized we were bonding. It worked on that trip as well as on subsequent occasions when visited our best friend. Identifying with a sponge had become everything, the big ticket. You begin to make adjustments to your "habits" even without knowing it; you go days without showering, your clothes are wrinkled and don't match, and the only thing that is important is sleeping. A friend of mine compared the first three months of raising a child to the eighth layer of hell.

RECOMMENDED READING

I am and probably always will be an avid reader; it is a great escape outside of watching taped episodes of *The Young and the Restless*. I read everything from lesbian romance to Native American literature to various fiction and nonfiction books. I highly recommend these books to prepare for the birth of your child, or simply for relief:

- *What to Expect When You're Expecting* (in very small doses; it can be very overwhelming). When you get to parts where they mention "father" or "dad," just substitute the non-pregnant partner and some stuff still applies. Hormonally and emotionally women are different creatures, whether you're pregnant or not; that is why I say "some stuff" applies.

- *The Three-Martini Playdate.* This book helped me understand that I didn't have to take everything so seriously.

- *Perfect Madness.* I started this book before our baby was born, and finished it a few months later;

intellectually challenging and has some good messages.

- *Lesbian Parenting.* A "must-have" bible, for obvious reasons.

- *Families like Mine.* An incredibly insightful book. It's a little scary, thinking about everything your family could potentially face, although it is a good dose of reality. An overall excellent read.

- *Down Came the Rain.* Insight into postpartum depression and the overall courageous journey into the depths of the scary side of being a parent. Postpartum depression doesn't discriminate; lesbian parents are just as susceptible.

I strongly encourage that after you have inundated yourself with every possible parenting, gay parenting, and birthing book imaginable, you spend the last trimester reading things that you really enjoy. The baby is coming regardless of what you read at this point, so if reading is something you enjoy, read now. It will be awhile before you pick up a novel again. I was and still am a big fan of lesbian fiction, there are some very good writers out there, and they afford you the escape that you so desperately need at this point.

FROM A-Z

- Get a well-woman checkup. Schedule your appointment with the NPP (non-pregnant partner) so that she can attend with you; if you're single, and don't mind a close friend going, it's great for support. Ask the tough questions: am I healthy enough? Come out, come out, whoever you are. In other words, identify your family and parenting situation, ask for a referral to a fertility clinic that will work with your best interests, and keep their opinions about your lifestyle to the cafeteria or water cooler.

- Do something wild and crazy. I spoke earlier about all the "last times." Getting pregnant by insemination requires planning, so do something fun that you won't have the opportunity to do for a while. For example, I surprised my partner with a banana-yellow Mustang convertible for a rental car when we were on vacation instead of our traditional, budgetary, two-door economy car that required Fred Flintstone to operate. Go on a day trip or overnight trip to somewhere fun; there with a little homework you can find great airfares.

- Every clinic works differently; find out if they recommend back-to-back insemination days, or once-a-month inseminations according to your ovulation kit.

- Unless Franklin Covey is planning your delivery, have your bag packed WELL in advance.

DECIDING TO FIND OUT IF THERE ARE ADDITIONAL BIRTHS

Some labs allow inquiries as to how many pregnancies and/or births a certain donor's sperm contributed to. I think that this inquiry should be handled with caution. Once you receive your answer, there is no turning back and erasing the knowledge you have obtained. Maybe it doesn't matter; you're just curious. Take, for example, a couple that conceives a child and then calls the lab to report the birth—which, by the way, the physician usually handles—and decides to ask the question. You then discover that the sperm you used has also contributed to (with straight or gay parents) nine other births, therefore allowing you to draw the conclusion that you and your partner's child has nine other half siblings running around the country. Sperm banks go to great lengths to ensure that proximity is considered when releasing sperm; in other words, they try to make sure that within a certain range, there will be a reduced chance of your child's prom date being their half brother. The whole point of this is, do you really want to know how many half siblings your child has in the world that you will never know about or be able to locate, and your child won't either? I think partners should weigh this phone call heavily, decide to do it or not and why you want the information or don't want the information, and then put it to bed. Go read to your child and forget about it.

TREADMILL

Lesbian or not, your treadmill will become a clothes hanger, a towel drier, a place to put things. It happens a lot. You have a treadmill, and it is usually in the room that is now the nursery. Both you and your partner are committed to returning to your workout routine once the baby is born and a routine is established. In fact, while your partner is pregnant, you actually think this is achievable—the working-out thing. Good luck. I still haven't figured out exactly when I am going to have time to reacquaint myself with the machine. In fact, like most nurseries it becomes part of the décor, regardless of the theme. From Dora to *Blue's Clues*, the treadmill becomes fashionable in the nursery. Gaining weight by the hour and using the treadmill for 101 uses that are not in the manual have become realities. Maybe one day, when my child can speak, he will tell me to move it, and then maybe, just maybe, I'll have the time and energy to get back on it. So kiss it goodbye until your child is in college.

Dr. Seuss—*Red Fish, Blue Fish*

One evening my partner and I were giving our infant a bath and reading him a bath book, one of those books that you can get wet and it's like a Timex: it keeps on ticking. Anyhow, I was listening to my partner read to our child, a tender moment, when we came upon an awkward spot in the bath book. The following is an excerpt from Dr Seuss, *One Fish, Two Fish, Red Fish, Blue Fish*: "Some are sad. And some are glad. And some are very, very bad. Why are they sad and bad? I do not know. Go ask your dad." Okay, I love Dr. Seuss; I like the stories; and our child likes how sing-songy the stories are. However, we kind of stopped dead in our tracks, blankly stared at each other, and then quickly substituted a word, fearful that our then-six-week-old child was going to ask who his dad was. In reality, it took several months for us to figure our how to substitute the word, since he can't read, just to make ourselves feel better because he wouldn't be knocking at our bedroom door at 3 a.m. wanting to know who his dad was. So after weeks and literally months of substituting "mom" for "dad," which didn't rhyme and drove me crazy, my partner finally substituted "granddad"—now that works! If we had gone another route besides artificial insemination, in which we knew who the father was and our child knew who he was, and he was actively involved in his life, it would have totally been a different story. Just one angle.

NEED FOR ADULT CONVERSATION

I soon realized after reading several Dr. Seuss books a familiar pattern with my speech. It wasn't that I couldn't string two syllables together, that I am from a small Midwestern town, or that I had limited contact with the adult world. After *Too Many Daves*, *The Sneetches*, and *The Cat in the Hat*, I could no longer formulate sentences that didn't rhyme. I would even catch myself pausing at the end of the first sentence to make sure I could end the second sentence as Dr. Seuss would have liked. The need for adult conversation is imperative and necessary. For lesbians, our initial adult conversation usually surrounds, "So are you Mommy or Momma?" Although I can understand everyone's curiosity, we have several months to figure it out. What I would really like to talk about is the spike of gasoline prices, global warming, the spotted owl, or the butterfly fluttering its wings to affect tides half a world away. Yes, we need to gloat about our baby; we need to ask questions; we need to voice our good-intentioned mistakes. We want to hear about work gossip from our co-workers, learn who is sleeping with whom, and the latest lesbian drama.

THE FIRST THREE MONTHS

The first three months are the most rewarding and exhausting times you will ever experience. It does go very fast, so those that tell you that are not lying! You will eventually get some sleep because your baby will eventually get older. You will learn things about your partner that you never knew, regardless of how long you have been together. This is also the time in which the physical pain associated with the birth subsides and your partner may begin the mumblings of having number two. Believe me, when she first comes home, she will tell you in different languages and in creative ways that she will never do that again! How quickly memory fades after three months. Your baby will come first all the time and you will forget to even put each other number two. Relationships get challenging, communication gets tougher, self-esteems get whacked out, and self-doubt blossoms. Please remember that you have added one additional role to your relationship—that of mother to each other's child. You are still partners in life, lovers, and best friends. This is absolutely crucial to remember and critical to bring balance to the family while raising your child. I can't underscore the importance of couples' counseling, as this becomes an issue that cannot be addressed between the two of you. I also highly recommend taking time out to have dinner together or go for a walk. This is a great time to build trust with the grandparents; let them have some time with their grandchild and take care of your relationship.

www.ingramcontent.com/pod-product-compliance
Lightning Source LLC
Chambersburg PA
CBHW021238280526
45784CB00005B/2142